GOOD M...
TO...

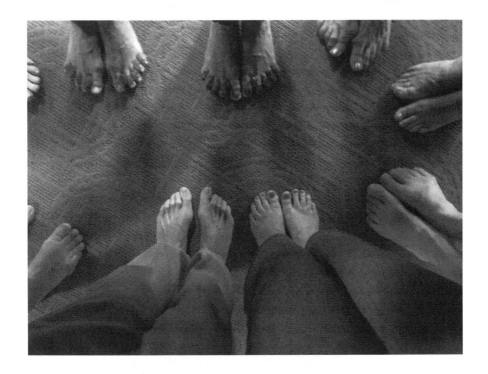

FEET WORK
for
CHAIR YOGA

Annette Wertman
2018

Good Morning Toes

A book of exercises for toes, ankles, feet and legs, to be used by yoga teachers and yoga students and chair yoga teachers and chair yoga students.

Copyright 2018-01-01

No part of this book may be reproduced, stored in a retrieval system or transmitted in any form or by any means, electronic, mechanical, photocopying, recording, scanning or otherwise without written permission of the author.

ISBN: 978-1976144738

Photographs by Annette Wertman & Glenn Coffin.

Cover design by Annette Wertman

Table of Contents

Introduction..5
  Why Keep Your Feet Healthy..7
Guidelines..8
  Chair Asana..9
  Feet in Chair Asana..10
  OM-Gratitude-Meditation..11
Pranayama
  Feel Your Breathing..12
  Angel Breath...13
Toe Work..14
  Toes Lift..15
  Scratching Yoga Mat..16
  Lift and Separate..17
  Foot Rolling..18
  Big Toe Lift...19
  Baby Toe Lift..20
  Middle Toes Lift..21
  Stretch & Squish..22
  The Foot Triangle...23
  Squish a Squash..24
  Washcloth Throw..25
  Toe Roll..26
Ankle Work...27
  Ankle Rotation..28
  Point & Flex... 30
  Outer Edge...31
  Inner Edge..32
  Inner & Outer Edge Both Feet..33
  Up On Toes...35
  Heel/Toe Rock..36
Knee Work..37
  Toe Crawl...38
  Knee Swing..39
  Foot Push...40
  Leg Extension..41
  Squats..42
Balance...43
  Up On Toes...44
  Knee Up..45
  Leg Back...46

Tree modified..47
  Tree..48
  Starfish..49
Benefits of Yoga Toes..51
  Regular Use...52

INTRODUCTION

"*Good Morning Toes*" (said out loud and all together!) is an interesting and unique way to begin a Chair Yoga class. Doing so engages the students and encourages a fun and relaxing atmosphere. But most importantly, saying "*Good Morning Toes*" brings awareness to Foot Health. Keeping our toes (feet) healthy and in the best condition possible is a worthwhile investment. The quality of our aging life depends on it!

   I have been teaching CHAIR YOGA privately and at community centres, neighbourhood houses, private residences and hospitals in Vancouver B.C. since 2010. Twice a year I spend 2 weeks at a resort (somewhere warm down south) teaching yoga to the guests of the hotel. I have seen a lot of toes and feet. Most of the toes and feet I see are NOT in such good condition! Unfortunately, this amazing structure (our foot) is highly underappreciated and therefore, undercared-for!

   This manual is a compilation of beneficial movements for toes, ankles, feet, knees and legs. I have also included balancing asanas (poses). Many of these movements are taken from other classes that I have attended. But many of the movements are the result of creative thinking in trying to fit the need. If you are a yoga teacher, explore these movements and learn how to instruct them with confidence and clarity. If you are a chair yoga student include the movements that are best for you, in your own home practice.

I encourage my yoga students to take off their shoes. Most do. Best to be able to freely move your toes and feel the ground beneath your feet. But, wearing socks is acceptable. Also, I do support the use of yoga toes.

I hope this manual helps in the need to stay strong and steady on your feet.

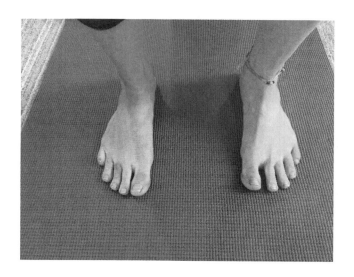

WHY KEEP YOUR FEET HEALTHY

Our feet connect us to the earth. They are our foundation and function as our base of support. 33 joints, 26 bones and 4 layers of arch muscle comprise this complex system that sends important messages to our brain. Our feet seem to be underappreciated until they cause problems. Common foot ailments such as weaken fallen arches, displaced deformed overlapping toes, planter fasciitis, claw toes, hammer toes, calluses and corns, bunions and swollen dark ankles, often cause knee problems, which can cause hip problems. Left untreated these problems can alter our body mechanics!

"When the foundation is weak or flawed problems arise. Many aches and pains – backaches, headaches, leg cramps, even a cranky disposition can be traced to the body's foundation – the FEET" * Suza

*The New Yoga for People Over 50' by Suza Francina

GUIDELINES

1. Use a sturdy, stable straight back chair, with a secure seat
2. Practice in a warm quiet place, without external distractions
3. Never force a movement or struggle with a pose
4. Pay attention and listen to your body. Only repeat movements as you are comfortable
6. Practice with bare feet (or appropriate socks)
7. Breathe consciously with each movement
8. Tell people, most importantly your health care practitioner, that you are practicing yoga
9. Be patient and enjoy your yoga practice
10. Use the chair to gain confidence and strength in balancing poses

CHAIR ASANA

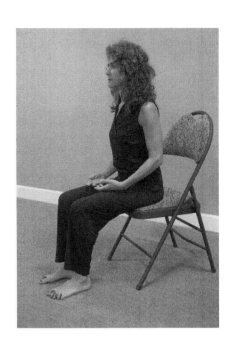

1. Sit tall at the edge of a sturdy stable chair
2. Feet flat on the floor, underneath your knees
3. Knees and feet two fists distance apart
4. Pull in your belly

FEET in CHAIR ASANA

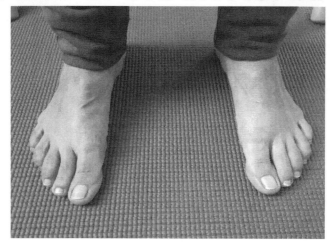

1. Keep feet parallel

2. Feel the floor

3. Push on your heels

OM - GRATITUDE - MEDITATION

1. Gently close your eyes
2. Slowly inhale to the count of 4
3. Exhale chanting OM. Repeat 2 more times
4. Chant: "May all beings be happy & free and may the happiness and freedom of my life contribute in some way to the happiness and freedom of all beings " *(Lokah Samasta Sukino Bavantu)*
5. Sit in stillness for a few minutes
6. Focus on your breath
7. Breathe deeper, smoother, and slower with each breath
8. Try to let your breathing relax you

PRANAYAMA

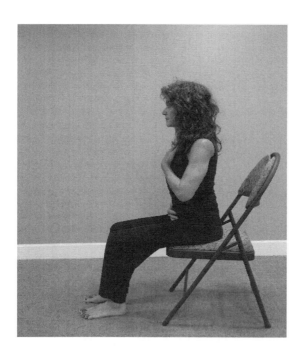

Feel your breathing

1. Hand on chest
2. Hand on belly
3. Hands on rib cage

ANGEL BREATH

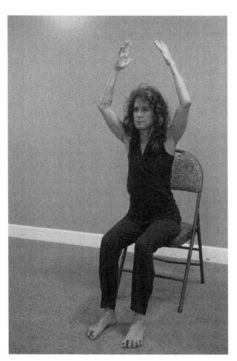

1. Sit tall at the edge of the chair
2. Press feet firmly into the floor and relax your shoulders
3. Inhale and slowly raise your arms above your head
4. Reach up
5. Exhale and slowly bring your arms down
6. Repeat a few times

TOE WORK

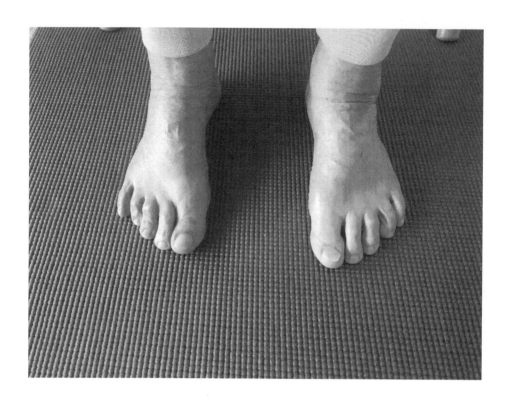

1. Toes Lift

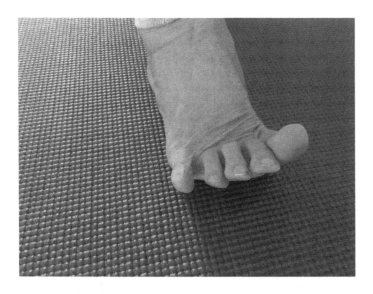

1. Stand in mountain pose (Tadasana) behind or beside a sturdy chair, or sit on the edge of a sturdy chair, with your feet parallel and about hip width apart
2. Stand/sit in silence. Find stillness and become aware of your breath
3. Inhale and exhale with each movement
4. Take 3 breaths as you just look at your toes
5. As you inhale lift the toes of the right foot, as you exhale place them back down. Do this 2 or 3 more times
6. Repeat same as above with your left toes
7. Try lifting all the toes of both feet, at the same time
8. Relax both feet and notice the feeling in your toes. Take 2 cleansing breaths

2. Scratching Yoga Mat

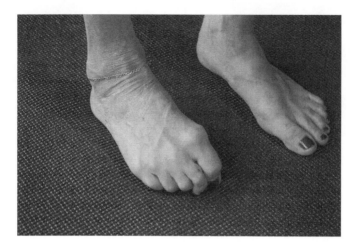

1. Stand in mountain pose (Tadasana) behind or beside a sturdy chair, or sit on the edge of a sturdy chair, with your feet parallel and about hip width apar
2. Stand or sit in silence. Find stillness and become aware of your breath
3. Inhale and exhale with each movement
4. Take 3 breaths as you just look at your toes
5. As you inhale bend the toes of your right foot, scratching the floor or your yoga mat. Exhale as you straighten your toes. Do this 4 or 5 more times
6. Repeat same as above with your left toes
7. Try this scratching motion with both feet (all your toes) at the same time
8. Relax both feet and notice the feeling in your toes. What did you experience?

3. Lift and Separate

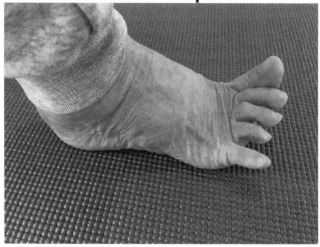

1. Stand in mountain pose (Tadasana) behind or beside a sturdy chair, or sit on the edge of a sturdy chair, with your feet parallel and about hip width apart
2. Stand or sit in silence. Find stillness and become aware of your breath
3. Inhale and exhale with each movement
4. Take 3 breaths as you just look at your toes
5. As you inhale lift and separate the toes of your right foot, stretching them apart. Exhale as you place your toes back down. Do this 4 or 5 more times
6. Repeat same as above with your left toes
7. Try this lifting and separating motion with both feet (all your toes) at the same time. Do this 4 or 5 more times

4. Foot Rolling

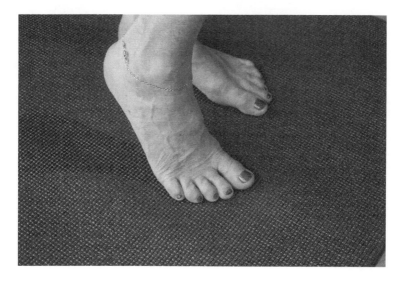

1. Stand or sit in silence. Find stillness and become aware of your breath
2. Take 3 breaths as you just look at your feet
3. Begin with the right foot (if standing shift weight to left foot). Inhale as you roll your foot up onto your toe tips, pressing them firmly
4. Exhale as you bring your foot back to flat, pushing on the heel. Repeat 3 to 5 times.
5. Inhale and roll on outside of foot, exhale bringing foot flat. Repeat 3 to 5 times
6. Inhale and roll on inside of foot, exhaling bringing the foot flat. Repeat 3 to 5 times
7. Repeat the entire sequence using your left foot
8. Relax and notice

5. Big Toe Lift

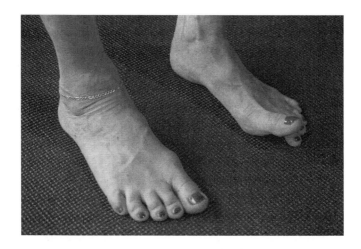

1. Stand in mountain pose (Tadasana) behind or beside a sturdy chair, or sit on the edge of a sturdy chair, with your feet parallel and about hip width apart
2. Stand or sit in silence. Find stillness and become aware of your breath
3. Inhale and exhale with each movement
4. Take 3 breaths as you just look at your feet
5. Feel equal weight on both feet. Begin with the right foot. Inhale as you lift up your big toe. Try pushing the other toes down at the same time
6. Exhale as you bring your big toe back down. Relax your toes
7. Repeat 3 to 5 times. Repeat the entire sequence using your left foot
8. Relax both feet and notice how you feel

6. Baby Toe Lift

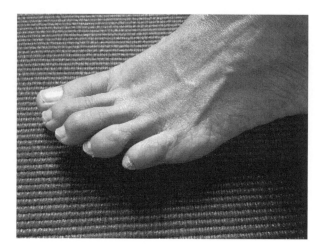

1. Stand in mountain pose (Tadasana) behind or beside a sturdy chair, or sit on the edge of a sturdy chair, with your feet parallel and about hip width apart
2. Stand or sit in silence. Find stillness and become aware of your breath
3. Inhale and exhale with each movement
4. Take 3 breaths as you just look at your feet
5. Feel equal weight on both feet. Begin with the right foot. Inhale as you lift up your baby toe. Try pushing the other toes down at the same time
6. Exhale as you bring your baby toe back down. Relax your toes
7. Repeat 3 to 5 times
8. Repeat the entire sequence using your left foot

7. Middle Toes Lift

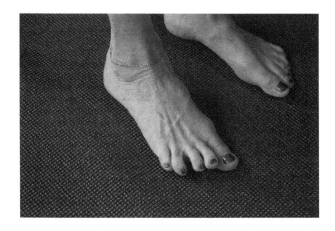

1. Stand in mountain pose (Tadasana) behind or beside a sturdy chair, or sit on the edge of a sturdy chair, with your feet parallel and about hip width apart
2. Stand or sit in silence. Find stillness and become aware of your breath
3. Inhale and exhale with each movement
4. Take 3 breaths as you just look at your feet
5. Feel equal weight on both feet. Begin with the right foot. Inhale as you lift up your middle toes Try pushing your big toe and baby toe down at the same time
6. Exhale as you bring your middle toes back down. Relax your toes
7. Repeat 3 to 5 times
8. Repeat the entire sequence using your left foot.
9. Relax both feet and become aware of the feeling in your toes

8. Stretch & Squish

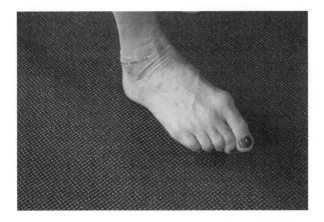

1. Stand in mountain pose (Tadasana) behind or beside a sturdy chair, or sit on the edge of a sturdy chair, with your feet parallel and about hip width apart
2. Stand or sit in silence. Find stillness and become aware of your breath
3. Inhale and exhale with each movement
4. Take 3 breaths as you just look at your feet
5. Begin with the right foot (if standing shift weight to left foot). Inhale as you stretch your toes apart
6. Exhale as you squish your toes together Repeat 3 to 5 times
7. Repeat the entire sequence using your left foot
8. Relax both feet and become aware of the feeling in your toes. Take 2 cleansing breaths
9. Take 2 cleansing breaths

9. The Foot Triangle

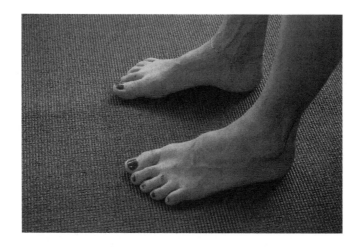

1. Stand in mountain pose (Tadasana) behind or beside a sturdy chair, or sit on the edge of a sturdy chair, with your feet parallel and about hip width apart
2. Stand or sit in silence. Find stillness and become aware of your breath
3. Inhale and exhale with each movement
4. Take 3 breaths as you just look at your feet
5. Begin with the right foot (if standing shift weight to left foot). Inhale as you feel the foot triangle: push down on the big toe, little toe and heel evenly
6. Exhale as you release. Repeat 3 to 5 times
7. Repeat the entire sequence using your left foot
8. Relax both feet and become aware of the feeling in your toes
9. Take 2 cleansing breaths

10. Squish a Squash

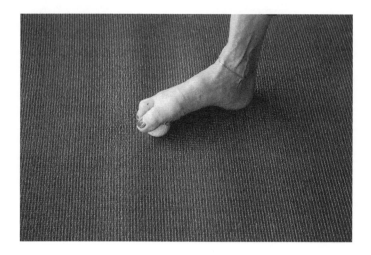

1. Stand in mountain pose (Tadasana) behind or beside a sturdy chair, or sit on the edge of a sturdy chair, with your feet parallel and about hip width apart
2. Stand or sit in silence. Find stillness and become aware of your breath
3. Inhale and exhale with each movement
4. Take 3 breaths as you just look at your feet
5. Begin with the right foot (if standing shift weight to left foot). Inhale as you squish a squash ball (or a golf ball) under your toes
6. Exhale as you release and relax your foot. Repeat 3 to 5 times
7. Repeat the entire sequence using your left foot
8. Relax both feet and become aware of the feeling in your toes

11. Washcloth Throw

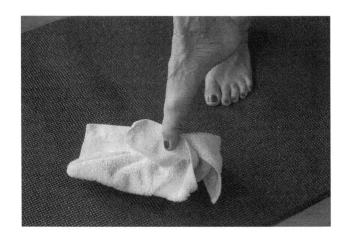

1. Stand in mountain pose (Tadasana) behind or beside a sturdy chair, or sit on the edge of a sturdy chair, with your feet parallel and about hip width apart
2. Stand or sit in silence. Find stillness and become aware of your breath
3. Inhale and exhale with each movement
4. Take 3 breaths as you just look at your feet
5. Begin with the right foot (if standing shift weight to left foot). Inhale as you pick up a washcloth using your toes
6. Exhale as you fling the washcloth to your neighbour
7. Relax your foot
8. Repeat using your left foot
9. Repeat this sequence a few times
10. Notice the feeling in your toes

12. Toe Roll

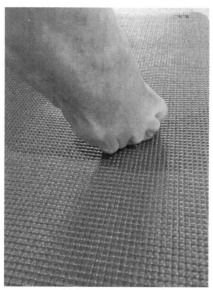

1. Stand in mountain pose (Tadasana) behind or beside a sturdy chair, or sit on the edge of a sturdy chair, with your feet parallel and about hip width apart
2. Stand or sit in silence. Find stillness and become aware of your breath
3. Inhale and exhale with each movement
4. Take 3 breaths as you just look at your feet
5. Begin with the right foot (if standing shift weight to left foot). Inhale as you point your ankle and gently roll over your toes
6. Hold for 3 to 5 breaths
7. Relax your foot
8. Repeat using your left foot.
9. Repeat this sequence a few times

Ankle Work

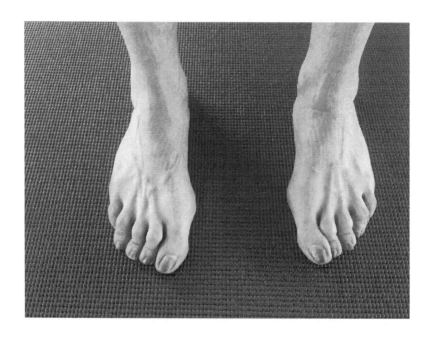

1. Ankle Rotation

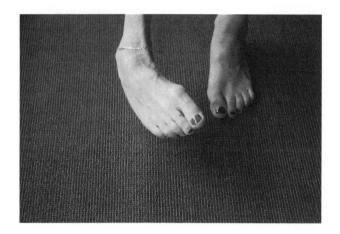

1. Stand in mountain pose (Tadasana) behind or beside a sturdy chair, or sit on the edge of a sturdy chair, with your feet parallel and about hip width apart
2. Your heels should be directly beneath your knees
3. Stand or sit in silence. Find stillness and become aware of your breath
4. Inhale and exhale with each movement
5. Take 3 breaths as you visualize or look at your ankles
6. Begin with the right foot (if standing shift weight to left foot)
7. Lift your right foot up, placing your hand under your knee. Interlace your fingers. In large slow circles rotate your ankle in one direction as you inhale
8. As you exhale, rotate in the other direction.
9. Repeat with same foot 2 more times. Gently place foot back down

10. Repeat rotations with left foot. Gently place left foot back down
11. Relax both feet. Be aware of the feeling in your ankles
12. Take 2 cleansing breaths
13. When foot is pointing down, point your toes
14. When foot is pointing up, separate your toes

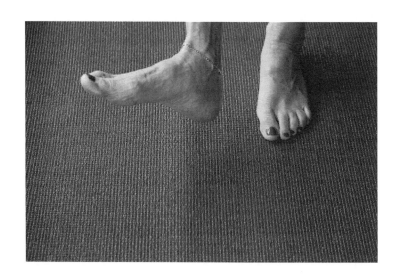

2. Point & Flex

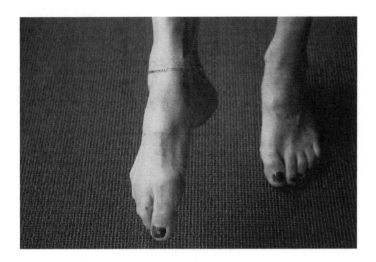

1. Stand or sit in silence
2. Your heels should be directly beneath your knees
3. Find stillness and become aware of your breath
4. Take 3 breaths as you visualize or look at your ankles
5. Begin with the right foot (if standing shift weight to your left foot)
6. Lift your right foot up, pointing your toes
7. Inhale as you slide your big toe along the floor to straighten your leg
8. Exhale and flex your foot, inhale pointing, exhale to bring your leg back
9. Repeat 3 to 5 times
10. Repeat these movements with left your foot
11. Relax both feet. Be aware of the feeling in your ankles

3. Outer Edge

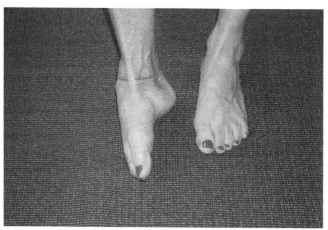

1. Stand in mountain pose behind or beside a sturdy chair, or sit on the edge of a sturdy chair, with your feet parallel and about hip width apart
2. Your heels should be directly beneath your knees
3. Stand or sit in silence. Find stillness and become aware of your breath
4. Inhale and exhale with each movement
5. Take 3 breaths as you visualize or look at your ankles
6. Begin with the right foot (if standing shift weight to left foot)
7. Shift your weight to the outer edge of your right foot
8. Inhale and exhale noticing the feeling. Flatten your right foot
9. Repeat 3 to 5 times
10. Repeat these movements with left your foot

4. Inner Edge

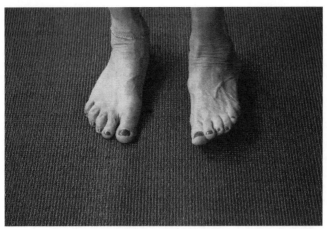

1. Stand in mountain pose (Tadasana) behind or beside a sturdy chair, or sit on the edge of a sturdy chair, with your feet parallel and about hip width apart
2. Your heels should be directly beneath your knees
3. Stand or sit in silence. Find stillness and become aware of your breath
4. Inhale and exhale with each movement
5. Take 3 breaths as you visualize or look at your ankles

   Begin with the right foot (if standing shift weight to left foot)
6. Shift your weight to the inner edge of your right foot
7. Inhale and exhale noticing the feeling. Flatten your right foot
8. Repeat 3 to 5 times
9. Repeat these movements with left your foot

5. Inner & Outer Edge Both Feet

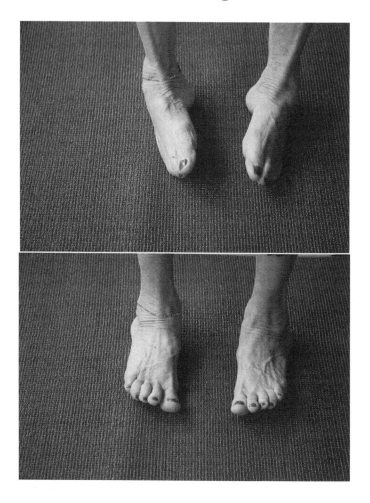

1. Stand in mountain pose (Tadasana) behind or beside a sturdy chair, or sit on the edge of a sturdy chair, with your feet parallel and about hip width apart
2. Your heels should be directly beneath your knees
3. Stand or sit in silence. Find stillness and become aware of your breath
4. Inhale and exhale with each movement

5. Take 3 breaths as you visualize or look at your ankles
6. Shift your weight to the inner edges of both feet.
7. Inhale and exhale noticing the feeling. Flatten both feet
8. Repeat 3 to 5 times
9. Repeat these movements shifting your weight to the outer edges of both feet
10. Relax both feet. Be aware of the feeling in your feet
11. Take 2 cleansing breaths

6. Up On Toes

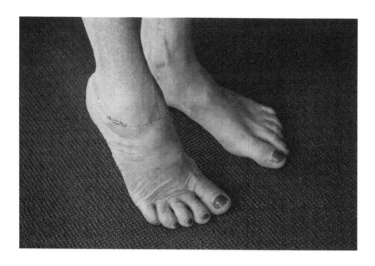

1. Stand in mountain pose (Tadasana) behind or beside a sturdy chair, or sit on the edge of a sturdy chair, with your feet parallel and about hip width apart
2. Your heels should be directly beneath your knees
3. Inhale and exhale with each movement
4. Take 3 breaths as you visualize or look at your ankles
5. Lift up right heel and push on the ball of the right foot
6. Exhale gently returning the heel to the floor
7. Repeat 3 to 5 times
8. Repeat these movements with your left foot
9. Repeat these heel lifts with both feet at the same time. Relax both feet

7. Heel/Toe Rock

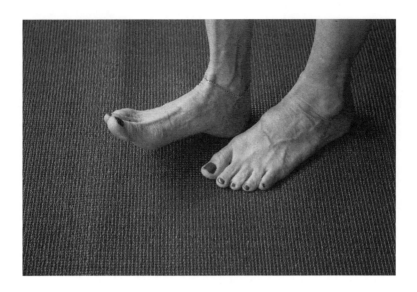

1. Stand or sit in silence. Find stillness and become aware of your breath
2. Inhale and exhale with each movement
3. Take 3 breaths as you visualize or look at your ankles
4. Inhale lifting up right heel and push on the ball of the right foot
5. Exhale gently returning the heel to the floor, lifting your toes
6. Repeat this rocking motion 3 to 5 times
7. Repeat these movements with your left foot
8. Repeat the heel/toe rock with both feet at the same time
9. Relax both feet. Be aware of the feeling in your feet

Knee Work

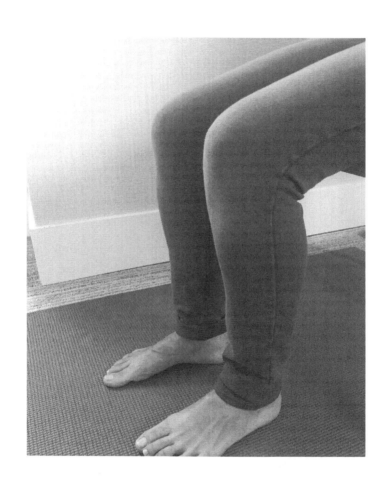

1. Toe Crawl

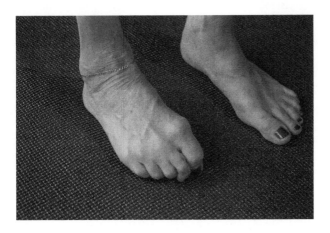

1. Stand in mountain pose (Tadasana), behind or beside a sturdy chair, or sit on the edge of a sturdy chair, with your feet parallel and about hip width apart
2. Your heels should be directly beneath your knees
3. Stand or sit in silence. Find stillness and become aware of your breath
4. Take 3 breaths as you visualize or look at your knees
5. Inhale, crawling the toes of your right foot forward, straightening your knee as much as comfortable
6. Exhale and notice the feeling in your knee
7. Inhale, crawling your right foot toes backwards bring your foot under your knee
8. Repeat these movements 3 to 5 times with your right leg. Repeat with left leg. Relax both feet

2. Knee Swing

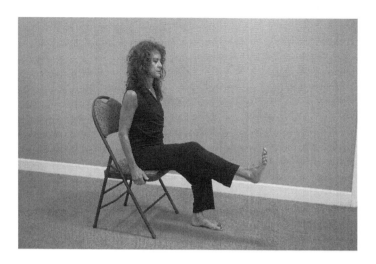

1. Stand in mountain pose (Tadasana) behind or beside a sturdy chair, or sit on the edge of a sturdy chair, with your feet parallel and about hip width apart
2. Your heels should be directly beneath your knees
3. Stand or sit in silence. Find stillness and become aware of your breath
4. Inhale and exhale with each movement
5. Take 3 breaths as you visualize or look at your legs
6. Inhale as you lift your knee; exhale as you extend your leg, keeping your foot flexed
7. Inhale as you bend your knee and exhale as you gently place your foot down
8. Repeat this gentle swing 3 to 5 times with same leg. Repeat with left leg

3. Foot Push

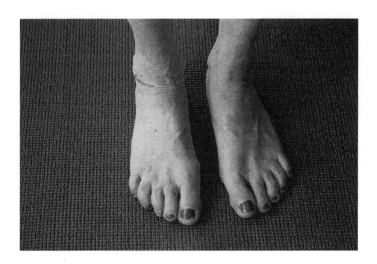

1. Stand in mountain pose (Tadasana) behind or beside a sturdy chair, or sit on the edge of a sturdy chair, with your feet parallel and about hip width apart
2. Your heels should be directly beneath your knees
3. Stand or sit in silence. Find stillness and become aware of your breath
4. Take 3 breaths as you visualize or look at your feet
5. Inhale and exhale while you push on the floor with your right foot
6. Try to tighten your leg muscles
7. Repeat this foot push 3 to 5 times
8. Repeat these movements 3 to 5 times with your left foot
9. Relax both feet. Be aware of the feeling

4. Leg Extension

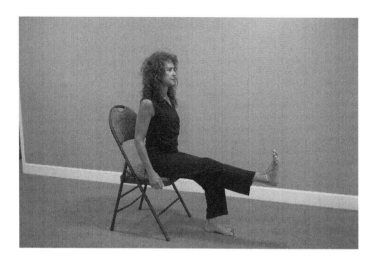

1. Stand or sit in silence. Find stillness and become aware of your breath
2. Inhale and exhale with each movement
3. Take 3 breaths as you visualize or look at your legs
4. Lift up your right foot so your heel is up off the floor and your right toe is touching the floor
5. Inhale, swinging your right leg forward as straight as comfortable. Flex your foot
6. Exhale swinging your leg back to a bent knee position
7. Repeat this swing 3 to 5 times
8. Repeat these movements 3 to 5 times with your left leg
9. Relax both feet
10. Repeat holding the leg extension
11. Be aware of the feeling in your legs

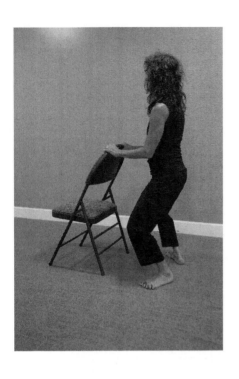

5. Squats

1. Stand in mountain pose (Tadasana) behind or beside a sturdy chair with your feet parallel and about hip width apart
2. Stand in silence. Find stillness and become aware of your breath
3. Inhale and exhale with each movement
4. Step your legs apart. Angle your feet out about 45 degrees
5. Hold on to the chair back or place your hands on your hips
6. Keeping your shoulders above your hips bend your knees slowly to a comfortable position
7. Exhale raising yourself up to straight legs
8. Repeat 3 to 5 times
9. Bring your legs back to hip distance apart

Balance

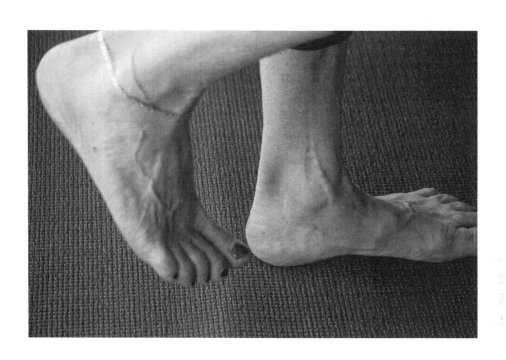

1. Up On Toes

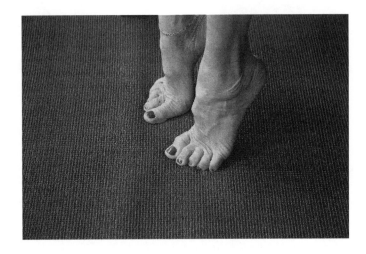

1. Stand in mountain pose (Tadasana) behind or beside a sturdy chair with your feet parallel and about hip width apart
2. Stand in silence. Find stillness and become aware of your breath
3. Inhale and exhale with each movement
4. Lift both heels standing up on your toes as high as comfortable
5. Hold on to the chair back or place your hands on your hips. Set your gaze (drishti)
6. Keep your shoulders above your hips
7. Exhale lowering your heels gently to the floor
8. Repeat this movement 3 to 5 times
9. Try staying up on your toes for a few seconds
10. Try closing your eyes

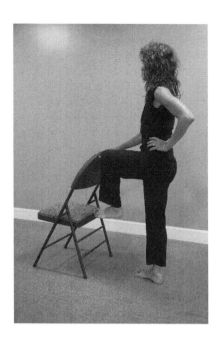

2. Knee Up

1. Stand in mountain pose (Tadasana) behind or beside a sturdy chair with your feet parallel and about hip width apart
2. Stand in silence. Find stillness and become aware of your breath
3. Hold on to the chair back or place your hands on your hips. Find your drishti
4. Keeping your shoulders above your hips, shift your weight to your left leg
5. Exhale lowering your leg gently to the floor
6. Repeat this movement 3 to 5 times
7. Try to stay with knee raised for 3 to 5 breaths
8. Repeat this movement with your left knee
9. Bring your legs back to hip distance apart
10. Be aware of the feeling in your ankles, knees and legs

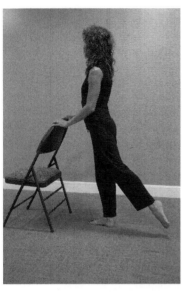

3. Leg back

1. Stand in mountain pose (Tadasana) behind or beside a sturdy chair with your feet parallel and about hip width apart
2. Stand in silence. Find stillness and become aware of your breath
3. Hold on to the chair back or place your hands on your hips. Set your gaze
4. Keeping your shoulders above your hips
5. Shift your weight to your left leg
6. Inhale sliding your right foot back behind you.
7. Point your right foot
8. Exhale lifting your right toe up about 2 inches from the floor. Keep leg back
9. Stay with foot raised for 3 to 5 breaths
10. Lower right foot gently to the floor and back beside left foot
11. Repeat this movement with left foot

4. Tree - modified

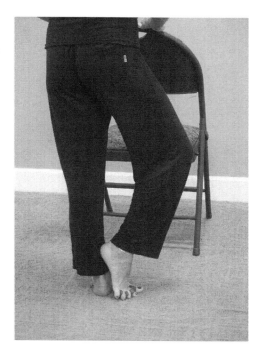

1. Stand in mountain pose (Tadasana) behind or beside a sturdy chair with your feet parallel and about hip width apart
2. Stand in silence. Find stillness and become aware of your breath
3. Hold on to the chair back or place your hands on your hips. Find a drishti
4. Keep your shoulders above your hips
5. Shift your weight to your left leg
6. Inhale sliding your right foot to a kick stand position
7. Stay in balance for 3 to 5 breaths
8. Lower right foot gently to the floor and back beside left foot
9. Repeat this movement with left foot, balancing on right leg

5. Tree

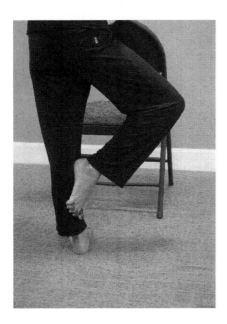

1. Stand in Tadasana holding on to the chair with right hand
2. Shift weight into left foot pressing evenly and firmly into the floor
3. Bend right knee and place the sole against the inner calf
4. Toes point towards the floor
5. Press the right foot into the right leg with equal pressure
6. Lengthen tailbone towards the floor
7. Find your drishti and gaze softly
8. When you feel steady raise your left arm over your head (maybe both arms up)
9. Reach entire body upward and breathe evenly
10. Relax shoulders, neck and face
11. With an exhalation step back to Tadasana
12. Repeat on other side

6. Starfish

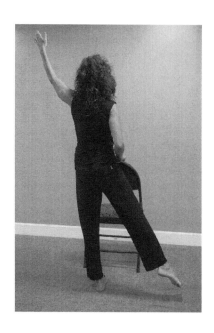

1. Stand in mountain pose (Tadasana) behind or beside a sturdy chair with your feet parallel and about hip width apart
2. Your heels should be directly beneath your knees
3. Stand in silence. Find stillness and become aware of your breath
4. Inhale and exhale with each movement
5. Hold on to the chair back or place your hands on your hips. Find your drishti
6. Keep your shoulders above your hips
7. Shift your weight to your left leg
8. Inhale sliding your right foot sideways
9. Point your right foot
10. Exhale lifting your right toe up about 2 inches from the floor. Keep leg as straight as possible
11. Stay with foot raised for 3 to 5 breaths

12. Raise left arm up and sideways, to create a diagonal stretch from toe to fingertip
13. Lower right foot gently to the floor
14. Lower left hand to the chair back
15. Repeat this movement with left foot and right arm

Benefits - Yoga Toes

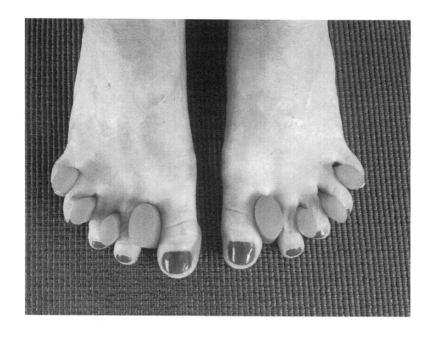

relax and rejuvenate tired, achy and swollen feet

increase foot strength and toe & ankle flexibility

stimulate circulation in your legs

stretch Achilles tendons

stretch leg muscles and improve arches

realign bones and soft tissue

correct postural alignment

prevent or help heal varicose veins, bunions & hammer toes

passive exercise for DVT (Deep Vein Thrombosis)

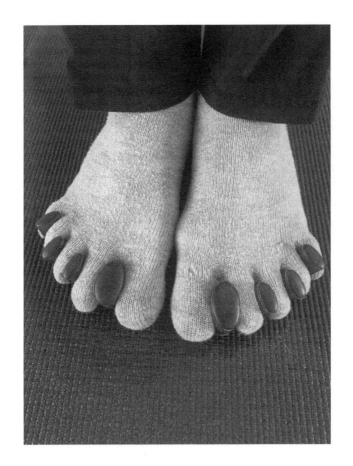

When you put your feet into a pair of **Yoga Toes**, you'll immediately notice the lifting and spreading of the toes, which stretches the muscles and Achilles tendon and stimulates the nerves and connective tissue.

Regular use *helps in healing conditions brought about by poor circulation, misalignment and lack of proper exercise.*

GOOD MORNING TOES

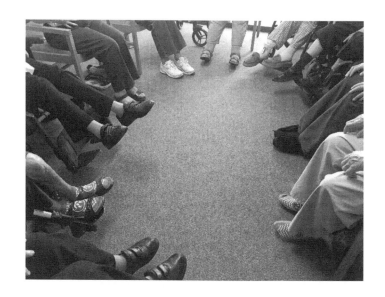

FEET WORK for CHAIR YOGA

Annette Wertman
2018

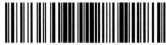

Printed in Poland
by Amazon Fulfillment
Poland Sp. z o.o., Wrocław